52 Weeks of Food for the Soul

Delicious Gluten-Free Recipes, Tasty Tips and Affirmations for Living a Healthy Lifestyle

Freddi Pakier CHC, AADP

ISBN 10:0692441107

Pakier Publishing
San Marcos, California

FreddiPakier.com

DEDICATION

This book is dedicated to all the magnificent women in my life who love to cook....my grandmother, Rachel Warszauer, who created beauty in everything she did; my mother, Lila Pakier, who was a gracious hostess and created works of art with the taste and presentation of her food; my sister, Idesa Pakier, who just recently tapped into her cooking talent; my daughters Stacy Kaplan and Lori Riegel who are both such creative and delicious cooks in addition to writing food blogs; my granddaughter Logan Riegel who not only bakes so beautifully but also creates magnificent food presentations; my granddaughter Sarah Kaplan who has become a very adventurous diner; and the first boy in our family, my grandson Joshua Kaplan who loves to eat, so it's fun for us to cook for him!

and to

Everyone who has ever said to themselves:

"I would like to obtain or maintain vibrant health through cooking simple, quick and easy recipes without dieting, ending 'yo-yo' dieting and knowing which foods are most important to eat."

ACKNOWLEDGEMENTS

It takes a village to birth a book. My first thanks goes to all of the students who have attended my cooking classes or participated in cleanses, many of which asked me "When will you write a book?"

Creating *"52 weeks of Food for the Soul"* would not have been possible without the support and help of so many people. My gratitude to the talented Judith Balian who designed the book's cover; she provided patient, dedicated support and shared her knowledge freely, with contributions to overall design, layout, and graphics.

To my friend, Jan Cormany, who was a student at my very first cooking classes years ago; who said "yes" to sharing her talent as a gifted editor.

A big THANK YOU to all of my recipe testers: Katherine Backman, Patricia Burke, Karen Christian, Jan Cormany, Brenda Ducloux, Joyce Gerber, Amy Krauss, Kathy Marinelli, Karen Overton, Teri Saisho, Lee Surwit, Laura Wilson, and Paula Yates. Your cooking and input were important in assuring that the recipes were tasty and easy to produce.

To Katherine Backman, Judith Balian, Brenda Ducloux, Allen Krauss, Nancy Link, Karen Overton and Teri Saisho for their encouragement, friendship and support.

And to my very special family: my sister, Idesa, who has been a constant source of loving support; to my daughters, Stacy and Lori, for putting up with me being busy all the time, and to my granddaughters Logan and Sarah and grandson, Joshua for bringing me joy.

DISCLAIMER

I am not a degreed medical doctor, dietitian or nutritionist. I make no claim to any specialized medical training, nor do I dispense medical advice or prescriptions. This content is not intended to diagnose or treat any disease. All content is based on my personal knowledge, opinions, and experience as a holistic health coach. It is intended to be provided for informational, educational and self-empowerment purposes ONLY. Please consult with your doctor or wellness team if you have questions regarding this whole foods program, and then make your own well-informed decisions based upon what is best for your unique genetics, culture, conditions, and stage of life.

CONTENTS

Quinoa or Buckwheat Stuffed Peppers 101
Super Salmon Salad 103
Tempeh "Chicken" Salad 109

SIDE DISHES
Beets with Mustard Dressing   27
Sautéed Brussels Sprouts with Kale 33
Cabbage Slaw with Apples and Walnuts 35
Daikon Quinoa Detox Salad 57
Shredded Brussels Sprouts with Lemon & Garlic 67
Kale Salad with Avocado and Capers   77
Kelp Noodles with Sautéed Greens 79
Roasted Root Vegetable Salad 91
Southwestern Quinoa Salad   93
Spinach, Beet and Orange Salad 105

DRESSINGS AND SAUCES
Basic Detoxifying Salad Dressing   19
Cranberry Raspberry Sauce   53
Orange Salad Dressing   61

DESSERTS
Honey Almond Cake 15
Chocolate Mousse 23
Chia Pudding 39
Baked Pears   45
Chocolate Bark   47
Chocolate Coconut Cookies   49
Oatmeal Raisin Flax Seed Cookies 65

BREAKFASTS
Blueberry Muffins 29
Avocado Kale Coconut Detoxifying Smoothie 51
Egg Muffins 59
Blueberry Green Tea Smoothie 73

"The way you think, the way you behave, and the way you eat, can influence your life by 30 to 50 years."

\- Deepak Chopra

INTRODUCTION

"Let food be your medicine and medicine be your food." - **Hippocrates**

As a drugless practitioner, my philosophy is the same as Hippocrates. Yes, food is our best medicine and this book is written for men and women who wish to achieve vibrant health through cooking these simple, quick and easy recipes in concert with positive thinking and actions towards wellness.

In my years of practice as a Holistic Health Coach I have learned from my clients that our health challenges are not just due to the lack of knowledge regarding what to eat, but also from internal messages and negative self-talk that sometimes sabotage creating the life we desire. So included in this book are 52 affirmations to practice for creating the health and weight we desire. As Deepak Chopra states, "What we think about, we become".

Our thoughts about food and our relationship with food develop when we are children. As a child of Holocaust survivors, food was an important item in our household. Eating was something very *serious*, which is probably an unusual word to use in thinking about food. My mother, who was a wonderful cook, served us very large portions of food and my Dad's statement when we sat down for a meal was; "Now it's time to eat." In other words, it wasn't time to talk, but to eat. My sisters and I were part of the "Eat Everything on Your Plate" family.

Still to this day, I always feel that if I don't have leftovers when I have guests for a meal that I didn't prepare enough food. We each have our own story and relationship with food and that informs what decisions we make about it.

HOW TO USE THIS BOOK

You can decide how to use this book. Perhaps you like order and will start at the beginning and add a food, affirmation and recipe to your wellness each week. Alternately, you might enjoy randomly flipping to a page and finding an affirmation, ingredient and recipe. It might be your body telling you exactly what it needs.

The bottom line is....health is wealth. In my health coaching practice and cooking classes I am often asked about which foods and ingredients are the most important for maintaining good health and promoting weight loss, so I have created a cookbook that provides the nutritional benefits of 52 healthy foods with accompanying recipes.

Variety is important in eating, and recipes were selected to "surprise our cells". Just as you should vary your workout routine, you should not eat the same foods every day. I have intentionally used many of the ingredients in more than one recipe so that you can experience the different ways that they can be incorporated into your lifestyle. The healing properties of the spices mentioned in the book are cumulative and are most effective when used as part of your regular daily diet.

My wish is that you have some fun cooking these recipes, that you discover new foods to include in your diet, that you find the joy in positive thinking, and that your good health blooms! L'Chaim…to good health!

Let's Connect!
Check out the resources on my website, and subscribe to my newsletter. I'd love to hear from you!

FreddiPakier.com

freddi@cox.net

I am perfect, whole, and complete just as I am.

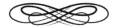

Almonds

✓ Great on-the-go snack when you're hungry

✓ Supply magnesium which is important for heart health

✓ Good source of calcium

✓ Contain vitamin E

✓ Supply potassium

✓ Provide fiber

✓ Good source of monounsaturated fat

✓ Provide eight grams of protein per ounce

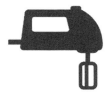

Honey Almond Cake

In my family, one of the foods that we served at the beginning of the New Year was honey cake. Honey is symbolic of creating sweetness in the New Year. Prior to healthier eating habits the cake was made with white flour as well as sugar. This version uses almond meal in place of flour so not only is it gluten-free but also provides protein.

Cake Ingredients

1 ¾ cups almond meal
4 large eggs, at room temperature, separated
½ cup honey
1 teaspoon vanilla extract
½ teaspoon baking soda
½ teaspoon salt
Topping Ingredients
2 tablespoons honey
¼ cup slivered almonds

Directions
Preheat oven to 350°F. Coat a 9-inch spring form pan with cooking spray. Line the bottom with parchment paper and spray the paper.

Beat 4 eggs in a large mixing bowl. Add remaining cake ingredients and mix until just combined. Scrape the batter into the prepared pan.

Bake until golden brown and a skewer inserted into the center comes out clean, about 25 minutes. Let cool in pan for 10 minutes. Run a knife around edge of pan and gently remove side ring. Let cool completely.

If desired, remove cake from pan bottom by gently sliding a large, wide spatula between cake and parchment paper. Carefully transfer cake to a serving platter. To serve, drizzle top of cake with honey and sprinkle with slivered almonds.

I am free of sugar cravings.

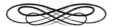

Apples

✓ Reduce cholesterol

✓ Decrease risk of diabetes from soluble fiber

✓ Can slow down plaque build-up

✓ Stimulate saliva production thereby lowering bacteria levels for healthier teeth

✓ Contain antioxidants

✓ Detoxify the liver

✓ Help control weight

✓ Have compounds that help reduce risk of cancer

✓ Prevent constipation

✓ Boost the immune system with quercetin

"Tomatoes and oregano make it Italian; wine and tarragon make it French. Sour cream makes it Russian; lemon and cinnamon make it Greek. Soy sauce makes it Chinese; garlic makes it good."

- Alice May Brock

Butternut Squash Apple Soup

Ingredients

4 cups butternut squash, peeled, seeded, cut in small pieces
3 medium sweet apples such as gala, chopped
2 cups onion, chopped
3 cups low sodium vegetable broth
2 teaspoons herbs de Provence or ½ teaspoon each: dried marjoram, thyme, and
    garlic powder and black pepper
Optional additions: 2 tablespoons almond or peanut butter or 1 can coconut milk

Directions

Combine the squash, apples, onion and vegetable broth in a large pot. Bring to a boil, then reduce heat, add herbs de Provence or marjoram, thyme, garlic powder and black pepper, and simmer uncovered for about 45 minutes, or until all vegetables are soft.

Using an immersion blender puree the soup (adding nut butter or coconut milk, if desired) and blend until smooth.   When ready to serve, heat again.

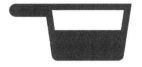

I am centered and relaxed, knowing every moment is an opportunity to give and to receive goodness.

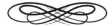

Apple Cider Vinegar

✓ Can kill bacteria and prevents it from reaching harmful levels

✓ Improves insulin sensitivity and helps lower blood sugar response after meals

✓ Increases feelings of fullness thereby helping with weight loss

✓ Has history of use as a disinfectant and natural preservative

"A fit, healthy body—that is the best fashion statement."
- Jess C. Scott

Basic Detoxifying Salad Dressing

Ingredients

1 tablespoon Dijon mustard
2 tablespoons lemon juice or organic apple cider vinegar
1 tablespoon olive oil

Directions

Wisk all ingredients in an empty salad bowl. Next add your greens, followed by vegetables, nuts, or fruits. Do not toss until ready to serve. Refrigerate if serving later. This is also a great way to transport salad to a gathering.

Serves 4 (Use one 5oz. bag of greens.)

All that I need to help me on my
healing path is here now.

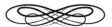

Asparagus

✓ Good source of fiber, vitamins A, C, E and K, as well as chromium, a trace mineral that enhances insulin's ability to transport glucose from the bloodstream into cells

✓ Loaded with antioxidants

✓ Contains folate which can prevent cognitive decline

✓ Contains glutathione, a detoxifying compound that helps break down carcinogens and free radicals

✓ Contains high levels of the amino acid asparagine, which is a natural diuretic

Asparagus Soup

6 Servings

Ingredients

2 medium potatoes, scrubbed and chopped
2 cups water
1 lb. fresh asparagus spears
2 cups shredded cabbage
1 cup loosely packed fresh parsley, chopped
¼ cup fresh basil, chopped
1 - 2 cups almond milk or other nut milk
¾ teaspoon salt, or to taste

Directions

Place potatoes in a large pot with 2 cups water. Bring to a simmer; cover and cook until tender when pierced with a fork, about 10 minutes. Remove tough ends from asparagus and cut into 1-inch lengths; should yield about 4 cups. When potatoes are tender, add asparagus, cabbage, parsley, and basil. Cover and simmer until asparagus is just tender, about 5 minutes. Use an immersion blender to purée soup while adding smaller amounts of almond milk to reach the desired consistency. Season to taste.

I take time for myself every day.

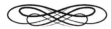

Avocados

✓ Rich in phytochemicals

✓ "Nature's butter"

✓ Provide heart-healthy monounsaturated fat

✓ 4 grams of protein

✓ Contain vitamin E and folate

✓ Have more potassium than bananas

✓ Contain fiber

✓ Can help moisturize dry skin and repair damaged hair

Chocolate Mousse

This is definitely a recipe that is not only easy to prepare but is healthy, guilt-free and delicious. Best of all, when you serve it to your guests they will be surprised to learn that this yummy dessert is made with avocado!

2 Servings

Ingredients
1 avocado, peeled and pitted
¼ cup cocoa powder
2 tablespoons honey
½ teaspoon vanilla extract
½ cup unsweetened vanilla almond milk

Directions
Combine all ingredients in a food processor and blend until well mixed and smooth. Chill in refrigerator for a couple of hours. Enjoy!

"All you need is love. But a little chocolate now and then doesn't hurt." - **Charles M. Schultz**

I listen to my body and feed it foods
that keep it healthy.

Beans

✓ High in antioxidants

✓ Contain fiber

✓ Contain protein

✓ Contain B vitamins, iron, magnesium, potassium, copper, and zinc

✓ May decrease the risk of diabetes, heart disease, and colorectal cancer

✓ Help with weight management

"We all eat, and it would be a sad waste
of opportunity to eat badly."
- Anna Thomas

Fennel, Tomato and White Bean Soup

This soup freezes well. If you prefer, you can add the spinach when reheating the soup. In my cooking classes and health coaching practice I always suggest cooking a pot of soup each week in a quantity larger than what you will eat that week. Freeze containers of a different soup each week and at the end of three weeks you will have a variety of healthy and delicious soups for quick and easy meals.

Makes 1 ½ quarts

Ingredients
1 tablespoon coconut oil
1 onion, diced
2 cloves garlic, minced
1 large bulb of fennel, thinly sliced
1 15oz. can of crushed tomatoes
4 cups of low sodium vegetable broth
1 15oz. can cannellini beans (white kidney beans)
5 oz. baby spinach
Salt and pepper to taste

Directions

Heat oil in a soup pot. Add onion, garlic, and fennel and sauté for 8-10 minutes or until the onion and fennel begin to look translucent.

Add tomatoes, broth, and beans and bring to a boil. Reduce the heat and simmer for 20-30 minutes. Before serving, stir in spinach and season with salt and pepper.

Health and happiness are my birthright,
and I claim them every day.

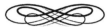

Beets

✓ Boost your energy

✓ Can lower blood pressure

✓ Can improve mental health

✓ Can help with weight loss

✓ Can help fight cancer

✓ Can reduce inflammation

✓ Used by the Romans as an aphrodisiac

✓ Can increase blood flow

✓ Are a great antioxidant

Beets with Mustard Dressing

Ingredients

4 medium beets
2 tablespoons lemon juice
1 tablespoon Dijon mustard
1 tablespoon apple cider vinegar
2 teaspoons maple syrup

Directions

Wash, and trim beets; steam over boiling water until tender, about 20 minutes. Remove from heat and while still warm, you can easily peel them. Slice into ¼ inch rounds. Whisk together lemon juice, mustard, apple cider vinegar and maple syrup. Pour over beets and toss. Serve hot or cold.

*Life flows through me easily
and comfortably as I allow change.*

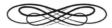

Blueberries

✓ Excellent laxative

✓ Blood cleanser

✓ Antioxidant

✓ Help prevent age-related mental decline

✓ Aid in reducing belly fat

✓ Help promote urinary tract health

✓ Improve digestion

✓ Help dissolve "bad cholesterol"

✓ Slow down visual loss

Gluten-Free Blueberry Muffins

Makes 12

Ingredients

3 cups almond meal
½ teaspoon sea salt
½ teaspoon baking soda
1 egg
1/3 cup coconut oil
2 tablespoons honey
1 teaspoon vanilla extract
1 cup blueberries, fresh if available

Directions

Preheat oven to 350 degrees. Line the muffin tin with paper muffin cups. Combine almond meal, sea salt and baking soda in a medium bowl and set aside. In a large bowl combine the egg, coconut oil, honey, and vanilla extract and whisk or beat on low with a hand mixer until well blended. Add almond meal mixture to wet ingredients blending well. With a rubber spatula gently fold the blueberries into the batter. Spoon about 2 tablespoons of batter into each paper-lined baking tin. Bake 17-20 minutes.

*I focus on being healthy because
what I focus on, I create.*

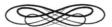

Broccoli

✓ Good source of calcium and protein

✓ Protects heart and blood vessels

✓ Can reduce cancer risk

✓ Can prevent osteoarthritis

✓ Provides lots of fiber

✓ Excellent source of vitamin C

✓ Good source of beta carotene, folate, chlorophyll, and magnesium

Broccoli Soup

Makes 2 quarts

Ingredients

1 onion, diced
1 tablespoon coconut oil
2 medium celery stalks, sliced
6 cups broccoli florets
1 ½ cups water
1 ½ cups almond milk
1 ½ teaspoons dried basil
½ teaspoon dried tarragon
Salt and pepper to taste

Directions

In a soup pot sauté onion in coconut oil until translucent. Add celery, broccoli, and water and bring to a simmer. Cover and cook over medium heat for about 10 minutes, Add almond milk, basil, and tarragon and heat for 5 more minutes. Blend with immersion blender and season to taste with salt and pepper.

Cooking is fun, quick and easy for me.

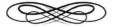

Brussels Sprouts

✓ Nutritious member of cruciferous family

✓ Good source of protein

✓ Contain iron and potassium

✓ Contains phytonutrients to fight disease

✓ Can boost immune system

✓ Contain vitamins A, B,C, K and omega-3's

✓ Supply us with fiber supporting colon health

✓ Contain calcium, magnesium, and potassium

✓ Reduce risk of heart disease with folate

Sautéed Brussels Sprouts with Kale

This is a favorite Thanksgiving recipe. I had the pleasure of taking cooking classes from Andrea Beaman (andreabeaman.com) when I was in New York City attending the Institute of Integrative Nutrition. Andrea shared this recipe in one of her newsletters many years ago.

Serves 2 to 4

Ingredients
2 tablespoons walnut oil
10-12 Brussels sprouts, cut in half
3-4 kale leaves, chopped into bite-sized pieces
1/3 cup water
1/4 cup dried cranberries
Sea salt
1/4 cup walnuts, roasted and chopped

Directions

In a sauté pan, heat walnut oil and add Brussels sprouts; sauté 3-5 minutes. Add kale, water, dried cranberries and a pinch of sea salt. Cover and cook on medium high heat for an additional 3-5 minutes or until kale is soft. Garnish with toasted walnuts.

*I give my body everything it needs to
bring it to optimal health.*

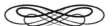

Cabbage

- ✔ Contains vitamin K and anthocyanin that help with mental function and concentration

- ✔ High in sulfur which helps dry up oily skin and acne

- ✔ Great for weight loss

- ✔ Helps detoxify the body

- ✔ Contains cancer preventive compounds

- ✔ Contains potassium which can help keep blood pressure low

- ✔ Has anti-inflammatory properties

"People who love to eat are always the best people."
- Julia Child

Cabbage Slaw with Apples and Walnuts

Serves 4 to 6

Ingredients

2 cups green cabbage, shredded
2 cups red cabbage, shredded
1 tablespoon apple cider vinegar
1/8 teaspoon fine sea salt
1/8 teaspoon ground black pepper
2 apples, cored and very thinly sliced
1/2 cup walnuts, toasted and chopped

Directions
In a large bowl, toss together green and red cabbage, vinegar, salt and pepper. Just before serving, add apples and walnuts and toss again.

Love surrounds, nourishes and protects me.

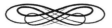

Cauliflower

✓ Can fight cancer

✓ Can improve blood pressure

✓ Contains anti-inflammatory nutrients

✓ Good source of vitamins C, B6, K, thiamin, riboflavin, niacin, magnesium, phosphorus, folate, pantothenic acid, potassium, and manganese

✓ Has fiber aiding in digestion

✓ Filled with antioxidants and phytonutrients to help body detoxify

✓ Good source of choline and vitamin B for brain health

Cauliflower and Sweet Potato Chowder

Makes 2 quarts

Ingredients

3 ¼ cups vegetable broth
4 large shallots, minced
½ cup celery, chopped
6 cups cauliflower florets (about 1 medium head)
1 cup chopped red bell pepper
1 medium sweet potato, peeled and cut into ½ -inch cubes (1 ½ cups)
1 bay leaf
1 cup unsweetened almond milk
2 tablespoons finely chopped fresh basil
Kosher salt to taste
Freshly ground black pepper to taste

Directions

Heat ¼ cup vegetable broth in a large saucepan over medium heat; add the shallots and celery and sauté for 5 minutes. Add the remaining 3 cups broth and 1 cup water; bring to a boil. Add the cauliflower, bell pepper, sweet potato, and bay leaf and bring to a boil. Reduce heat, cover, and simmer for 20 minutes. Remove the bay leaf. Remove from heat and add almond milk. For a heartier consistency, purée one half to all of the soup in batches using anblender or immersion blender. Add the basil and season with salt and black pepper.

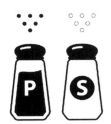

My energy expands with physical activity.

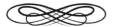

Chia Seeds

✓ 8 times more omega-3 than salmon

✓ 6 times more calcium than milk

✓ 3 times more iron than spinach

✓ 15 times more magnesium than broccoli

✓ Twice as much fiber as bran flakes

✓ A complete protein with 6 times more than kidney beans

✓ Cleanses and soothes the colon while supporting digestion.

✓ Provides long-lasting energy

✓ Source of vitamins A, B, D and E, and boron, copper, molybdenum, niacin, potassium, silicon, sulphur, thiamine and zinc

Chia Pudding

Quick and easy to prepare; a perfect treat if you miss sweets.

Ingredients

1 14oz. can of coconut milk
2-3 cups washed and stemmed strawberries (substitute frozen)
½ teaspoon vanilla extract
3 dates, pitted
pinch of sea salt
½ cup chia seeds

Directions

Combine all ingredients except chia seeds in a high speed blender and blend until smooth. Add chia seeds to liquid and refrigerator for at least one hour or overnight. Sprinkle with cinnamon if you like.

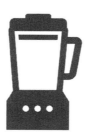

I monitor my self-talk and make sure it is uplifting and supportive.

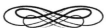

Celery

✓ Can reduce inflammation

✓ Contains magnesium which sooths the nervous system and keeps you calm

✓ Great for weight loss

✓ Can aid in digestion

✓ Can reduce "bad" cholesterol

✓ Contains vitamin A which helps protect the eyes

✓ Can lower blood pressure

✓ Contains pheromones that boost your arousal levels

Chicken Soup

Ingredients

1 3 lb. whole, organic chicken
4 carrots, sliced
4 stalks celery, sliced
1 large onion, diced
1 small bunch fresh dill, if desired
Salt and pepper

Directions

Place the chicken, carrots, celery, dill and onion in a large soup pot and cover with boiling water. Heat and simmer covered until the chicken meat is almost falling off of the bone; about 1 ½ hours. Skim off foam every so often.

Remove chicken from pot and separate meat from bones with a fork. Season broth with salt and pepper and return chicken to pot. Stir and serve.

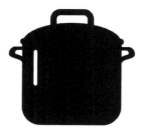

I radiate health.

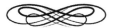

Cilantro

✓ Powerful natural cleansing agent for toxic metals

✓ Has a blood sugar lowering effect

✓ Has antioxidant properties

✓ Is a natural fungal cleanser

"You don't need a silver fork to eat good food."
                                    - Paul Prudhomme

Ginger and Cilantro Baked Cod

Serves 2

Ingredients

2 large cod fillets (or similar thin white fish) - about ¾ pound
3 garlic cloves, minced
1 inch piece of ginger - (1 tablespoon grated)
2 tablespoons Bragg's Liquid Aminos
1/4 cup white wine
1 teaspoon sesame oil
1/3 cup chopped cilantro
Scallions, chopped for garnish
Extra cilantro, to garnish

Directions

Heat the oven to 375°F. Pat the fish dry and season lightly with salt and pepper. Place in a glass baking dish.

Chop the garlic, and grate the ginger. Whisk together Bragg's Liquid Aminos, white wine, sesame oil, and cilantro. Add pepper, garlic and ginger and pour sauce over the fish, lightly rubbing into fish. Bake for about 12 minutes or until fish flakes easily and is cooked through. It will be very moist. Serve immediately over brown rice, garnished with scallions and cilantro.

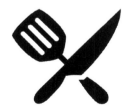

My kitchen is my wellness center.

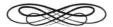

Cinnamon

✓ Regulates blood sugar

✓ Reduces "bad" cholesterol levels

✓ Contains natural anti-infectious compounds

✓ Is a natural food preservative

✓ Contains fiber, calcium, iron, and manganese

✓ Reduces arthritis pain

✓ Helps balance hormones

Baked Pears

Serves 4

Ingredients

4 pears (any type)
2 cups apple juice
1 cinnamon stick
6-8 cloves

Directions

Preheat oven to 400 degrees. Cut a thin slice off the bottom of each pear to help them stand upright in a baking dish. Pour apple juice into dish; add cinnamon stick and cloves. Roast pears for about 1 ½ hours, basting every 30 minutes, until tender, brown, and puckered.

Remove pears from oven and place on a serving platter. Drizzle the liquid from the bottom of the baking pan over the pears. They can be served warm or cold.

Sliced leftover pears are a wonderful addition to a green salad or mixed into Greek yogurt.

It feels good to be my optimal weight without dieting.

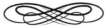

Dark Chocolate

✓ Can lower blood pressure

✓ Can reduce risk of heart attack and stroke

✓ Lessens craving for sweet, salty and fatty foods

✓ Reduces stress hormones

✓ Can help control blood sugar

✓ Boosts brain power

✓ Loaded with antioxidants.

✓ High in vitamins and minerals (potassium, copper, magnesium and iron)

"Seize the moment. Remember all those women on the Titanic who waved off the dessert cart."
— **Erma Bombeck**

Chocolate Bark

Ingredients

1 12 oz. bag chocolate chips with 6 grams or less of sugar
¾ cup nuts, seeds, or dried fruit of your choice (or a combo)

Directions

This is so simple! Just melt a bag of chocolate chips in a double boiler or in a bowl placed over boiling water. Mix in any ingredients that you would enjoy having in your bark. Spread on a waxed paper- lined cookie sheet and refrigerate for one hour or until firm. When firm, break apart and enjoy!

Variation: Spread chocolate on waxed paper and then sprinkle nuts, seeds or dried fruit on top. A great holiday combination is pistachio nuts and dried cranberries.

I balance my life between work, rest and play.

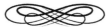

Coconut Oil

✓ Promotes heart health

✓ Promotes weight loss

✓ Supports your immune system

✓ Supports a healthy metabolism

✓ Provides you with an immediate energy source

✓ Keeps your skin glowing

✓ Supports the thyroid gland

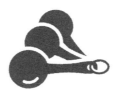

Chocolate Coconut Cookies

Makes 30 Cookies
Ingredients

2 cups unsweetened shredded coconut
1 cup almond meal
¼ teaspoon sea salt
½ cup coconut oil, melted
½ cup coconut palm sugar
1 teaspoon vanilla extract
¼ teaspoon almond extract
2 eggs, beaten

Chocolate Drizzle

¾ cup dark chocolate, 73% cocoa or higher
2 tablespoons coconut oil

Directions

Preheat oven to 300 degrees. Line a baking sheet with parchment paper. In a medium bowl combine the shredded coconut, almond flour and sea salt. In another medium bowl combine ½ cup melted coconut oil, coconut sugar, vanilla extract, almond extract and beaten eggs. Add the dry ingredients to the wet ingredients and mix. Form round, golf-ball sized balls with the dough. Place 2 inches apart on the prepared baking sheet.

Bake for 30 minutes, or until golden. Allow to cool for 20 minutes and then refrigerate for an additional 20 minutes.

Meanwhile, melt the chocolate and coconut oil in a double boiler or a bowl placed over boiling water. Mix constantly until smooth. Drizzle dark chocolate across the tops of the cookies. Return to refrigerator to harden the chocolate - about 15 minutes.

I think positive thoughts because
my thoughts determine my actions.

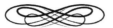

Coconut Water

✓ Aids in weight loss

✓ Hydrates the body by replacing potassium

✓ Helps reduce blood pressure

✓ Facilitates digestion

✓ Contains calcium, magnesium, phosphorous, and sodium which are the five essential electrolytes in the human body

✓ Clears up and tones the skin

Avocado Kale Coconut Detoxifying Smoothie

Makes 2 servings

Ingredients

1 ¼ cups coconut water
2 cups kale leaves
1 avocado
1 frozen banana
1 lemon, juiced

Directions

Pour coconut water into blender. Add kale, avocado, frozen banana and lemon juice. Blend until smooth. Pour into two glasses and serve immediately.

*Healing energy flows through every organ,
joint and cell in my body.*

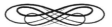

Cranberries

✓ High in vitamin C

✓ Have antioxidant and antibacterial effects in the body

✓ Rich source of the flavonoid quercetin which inhibits breast and colon cancer development

✓ Help maintain a healthy urinary tract

✓ Beneficial to the eyes - can help prevent cataracts, macular degeneration, and diabetic retinopathy symptoms

Cranberry Raspberry Sauce

When cranberries are in season I always buy a few extra bags to freeze for this quick and easy year-round cranberry dish.

Ingredients

1 bag (12-16 oz.) fresh cranberries
1 bag frozen raspberries
1-2 tablespoons maple syrup (optional)

Directions

Rinse cranberries with cold water in colander. Put in pot and pour in just enough water to reach the top of the cranberries. Bring to a boil and add bag of frozen raspberries. Turn heat to medium-low and cook until cranberries start to fall apart. Add maple syrup or additional sweetness if desired.

Leftover cranberry sauce is wonderful mixed into Greek yogurt.

I am awake and alert to wonderful, positive surprises.

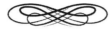

Curry

- ✓ Controls blood sugar
- ✓ Has cancer-preventive benefits
- ✓ Helps lower cholesterol
- ✓ Helps the body detoxify

Curried Cauliflower Soup

Ingredients

1 large head cauliflower, cut into florets
1 tablespoon curry powder
¼ teaspoon ground cumin
¼ teaspoon ground coriander
1/8 teaspoon ground cinnamon
6 cups vegetable broth (or less)
2 tablespoons coconut oil
1 tablespoon olive oil
Sea salt
1 cup yellow onion, diced
2 carrots, peeled and sliced thin
1 cup diced celery

Directions

Preheat oven to 400 degrees and line a baking sheet with parchment paper. Toss the cauliflower with 1 tablespoon olive oil and ¼ teaspoon sea salt; spread in even layer on the pan. Bake until the cauliflower is tender (about 25 min.).

While cauliflower is roasting, heat the coconut oil in a soup pot over medium heat. Add onion and sauté until translucent - about 3 minutes. Add the carrots and sauté until the vegetables begin to brown - about 12 minutes. Add the curry powder, cumin, coriander, and cinnamon and stir until the spices have coated the vegetables.

Add 5 cups vegetable broth and stir; heat for 5 minutes. Add the roasted cauliflower to the pot with the broth. Check for desired amount of liquid (adding more broth if needed) to assure a nice consistency when the soup is pureed. Use an immersion blender to puree the soup.

It is gratifying to share healthy meals with family and friends.

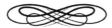

Daikon Radish

✓ Excellent source of fiber

✓ Contains vitamin C, phosphorous and potassium

✓ Contains natural enzymes that aid digestion of fat and carbohydrates

✓ Curbs sugar cravings

Daikon Quinoa Detox Salad

4-6 Servings

Ingredients

2 cups cooked quinoa
1 daikon radish, grated
2-4 carrots, grated
½ -1 cup micro greens (or baby greens)
½ bunch mint leaves, roughly chopped
1 avocado, diced
Handful of raw sunflower seeds
Juice of 1 lemon, or more to taste
Drizzle of olive oil
Sea salt and pepper to taste
Pinch of cayenne pepper

Directions

Combine all ingredients and serve.

I honor myself by selecting nutritious food and beverages.

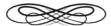

Eggs

✓ Rich source of choline in yolk -vital for optimum brain function and reduced inflammation

✓ Choline helps produce serotonin and dopamine (the happiness hormone)

✓ Choline contains lutein which protects against vision loss

✓ High in sulfur which supports liver function

✓ Egg yolks are a rich source of B-complex

✓ Contain sulfur which is necessary for the production of collagen and keratin which helps maintain shiny hair, strong nails and glowing skin

✓ Has highly digestible amino acids

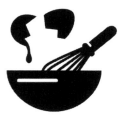

Egg Muffins

Makes 12

Ingredients

12 eggs
1 red bell pepper, diced
½ large yellow onion, diced
Salt and pepper to taste
Chopped fresh herbs of your choice

Directions

Pre-heat oven to 400 degrees. Crack eggs into a large bowl and whisk until fluffy. Stir in diced peppers, onions, and herbs, and season with salt and pepper. Coat a 12-cup muffin tin with cooking spray (or coconut oil) and evenly divide egg mixture in all 12-cups.

Bake muffins for 20 minutes or until the eggs are set. Do not overcook.

*I take care of myself physically,
emotionally, and spiritually.*

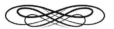

Extra Virgin Olive Oil

✓ High in antioxidants

✓ Contains vitamins E and K

✓ Anti-inflammatory

✓ High in monounsaturated fat

✓ Protects against heart disease

*"So, if I'm cooking, I'll be steaming vegetables,
making some nice salad, that kind of stuff."*
- Paul McCartney

Orange Salad Dressing

Ingredients

2 oranges, zested
Juice of 1 large orange
2 tablespoons balsamic vinegar
2 tablespoons honey
1 clove garlic, minced
Freshly ground black pepper and salt to taste
3/4 cup extra-virgin olive oil

Directions

Combine all ingredients in a jar with tight lid and shake to blend. Refrigerate to develop flavors.

Energy, enthusiasm and vitality are my birthright.

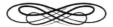

Fennel

✓ Contains essential oils which have anti-fungal and anti-bacterial properties

✓ Contains anti-oxidants

✓ Contains fiber

✓ Contains folic acid

✓ Contains vitamin C

✓ Contains potassium which helps reduce blood pressure

✓ Contains copper, iron, calcium, magnesium, manganese, zinc, and selenium

Roasted Fennel and Carrot Soup

Ingredients

2 medium fennel bulbs with fronds
1 pound carrots, quartered lengthwise
1 medium onion, quartered
1 garlic clove, peeled
3 tablespoons olive oil
½ teaspoon coconut sugar
2 ½ cups reduced-sodium chicken or vegetable broth
2 ½ cups water

Directions

Preheat oven to 450°F with rack in lowest position.

Chop enough fennel fronds to measure 1 tablespoon and reserve. Discard stalks and remaining fronds. Slice bulbs ¼ inch thick and toss with carrots, onion, garlic, 3 tablespoons oil, sugar, ½ teaspoon salt, and ¼ teaspoon pepper in a large bowl. Spread in a rimmed baking pan and roast, stirring occasionally, until browned and tender, about 25 to 30 minutes.

In a soup pot combine the broth and water. Add roasted vegetables and blend with an immersion blender, thinning to desired consistency with extra water. Simmer to heat and season with salt and pepper. Garnish with reserved fennel fronds.

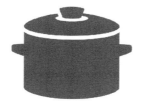

Taking good care of my health is like depositing money in the bank.

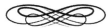

Flax Seeds

✓ Rich source of essential fatty acids and omega-3

✓ Protect against heart disease, cancer, and autoimmune diseases such as multiple sclerosis and rheumatoid arthritis

✓ Helps alleviate constipation and bloating

✓ Eliminates toxic waste

✓ Strengthens the blood

✓ Reduces inflammation

✓ Accelerates fat loss

✓ Reduces depression

Oatmeal Raisin Flax Seed Cookies

Ingredients

1-cup oatmeal, blended until flour-like or 1 cup oat flour
¼ cup flax seeds, blended until flour-like
1 14 oz. can cannellini beans, drained and blended until smooth
½ cup oatmeal
¼ cup flax seeds
½ cup raisins
½ cup applesauce

Directions

Preheat oven to 350 degrees. Mix all ingredients together. It should be a wet mixture. Scoop by tablespoon onto parchment lined baking sheet. Bake for 8-10 minutes.

Optional add-ins:
¼ cup pure maple syrup
Chocolate chips, nuts, or sesame seeds

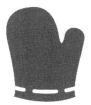

I take time to breathe deeply each day,
allowing my body to relax.

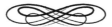

Garlic

✓ Stimulates the immune system

✓ Effective antibiotic and antiviral agent – a powerful natural medicine

✓ Can lower high blood pressure and cholesterol

✓ Can reduce the risk of cancer

"One cannot think well, love well, or sleep well, if one has not dined well."

- Virginia Woolf

Shredded Brussels Sprouts with Lemon and Garlic

Ingredients

3 cups shredded Brussels sprouts (you can buy pre-shredded sprouts)
1 tablespoon olive oil or coconut oil
2 cloves of garlic, chopped
Sea salt to taste
Pepper to taste
Squeeze of fresh lemon juice

Directions

Quickly sauté Brussels sprouts in oil with garlic for about 2 minutes over medium heat. Stop sautéing when they turn bright green. Add salt, pepper and lemon to taste. Serve immediately or refrigerate and eat cold.

To Shred Brussels Sprouts

Cut Brussels sprouts in half. Lay flat side down and cut across the sprout making little shreds.

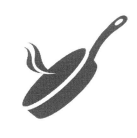

*I am kind and gentle with myself,
no matter what happens.*

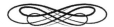

Ginger

✓ Lowers blood sugar, cholesterol, and blood fats

✓ Antibiotic and antifungal capability

✓ Anti-inflammatory properties

✓ Dulls appetite

✓ Ignites digestive juices

✓ Helps clear sinuses and congestion

✓ Helps overcome motion sickness and nausea

✓ Reduces flatulence and stomach cramps

✓ Aphrodisiac properties

✓ Improves absorption and assimilation of nutrients

Ginger Glazed Mahi Mahi

Ingredients

4 6oz. Mahi Mahi filets or another white fish
4 tablespoons Bragg's Liquid Aminos
1 tablespoon freshly grated ginger
2 garlic cloves, crushed
Salt and pepper to taste

Directions

In a small bowl mix the Braggs Liquid Aminos, ginger and garlic. Season fish with a little sea salt and pepper and place the filets in a baking pan. Pour glaze mixture over fish and bake at 350 degrees for 15 to 20 minutes until fish is cooked through. Optional: baste with pan liquid once half way through cooking time.

*I enjoy cooking because it helps me stay healthy
and maintain my ideal body weight.*

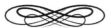

Greek Yogurt

✓ Contains calcium, potassium, phosphorus and magnesium

✓ Helps promote weight loss

✓ Contains vitamins vital for energy metabolism and the health
of neurological, immune and cardiovascular systems

✓ Contains live probiotic cultures which may help protect against
harmful bacteria

✓ Protein-rich and 2 times the protein of regular yogurt

Strawberry Yogurt Soup

2 Servings

Ingredients

1 pint washed strawberries, cut into bite size pieces (or 12 oz. frozen)
1/2 cup orange juice
1 teaspoon honey
½ teaspoon cinnamon
1 cup Greek yogurt

Directions

Combine strawberries, orange juice, honey and cinnamon in saucepan and heat until mixture begins to bubble (do not let it burn). Cool mixture for 10 minutes. Cover and refrigerate for 30 minutes. Pour strawberry mixture into blender or food processor and add yogurt. Puree until smooth. Serve garnished with mint leaves. (This recipe can be used to make delicious frozen pops.)

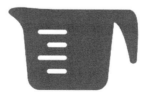

I practice loving myself and feel radiantly alive.

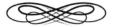

Green Tea

- ✓ Lowers cholesterol levels and the risk of heart disease

- ✓ Helps protect against bacterial infections

- ✓ Promotes joint health and stronger bones

- ✓ Reduces inflammation

- ✓ Provides mild stimulation and mental focusing effects

"A woman is like a tea bag - you can't tell how strong she is until you put her in hot water."
- Eleanor Roosevelt

Blueberry Green Tea Smoothie

Serves 2

Ingredients

2 green tea bags
2 cups frozen blueberries
1 ½ cups Greek yogurt
3 dates
½ teaspoon vanilla
2 teaspoons flax seeds
2 teaspoons chia seeds
¾ cup water

Directions

Bring water to boil; pour over tea bags and steep for about 4 minutes. Squeeze and remove tea bags, chill the tea overnight. Place all the ingredients in blender, process until smooth and divide the smoothie into ice filled glasses.

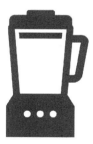

*I take the time to chew each bite of food
because digestion begins in the mouth.*

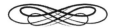

Hemp Seeds

✓ Excellent source of essential fatty acids including Omega-3s

✓ Contains Vitamin E

✓ Increases energy levels and metabolic rate

✓ Helps lower "bad" LDL cholesterol levels

✓ Helps lower blood pressure

✓ Supports immune system

✓ Helps reduce inflammation and the symptoms of arthritis

✓ More digestible protein than meat, eggs, or dairy

✓ Improves muscle recovery after exercise

✓ Improves organ function and cardiovascular circulation

✓ Reduce symptoms of PMS and menstrual cramps

Flourless Banana Bread

Gluten-free, grain-free, dairy-free, soy-free, paleo, and sugar-free!

My sister Idesa, who is very creative and talented, didn't discover her cooking and baking talent until she made this recipe for the first time when she was in her 60's. Now, not only does she make this when she has an oversupply of bananas, but she gets regular requests for it from friends. Instead of making it into bread, Idesa often pours the batter into muffin pans.

Ingredients

3 ripe bananas
½ cup almond or sunflower butter
3 eggs
3 tablespoons hemp seeds
3 tablespoons Chia Gel (mix 9 tablespoons of water with 3 teaspoons chia seed and let sit for 15-20 minutes. The chia seeds will puff into a gel.)
¼ teaspoon salt
1 teaspoon baking powder
1 teaspoon cinnamon
1 teaspoon vanilla extract
Optional: ½ cup chopped walnuts or ½ cup chocolate chips

Directions

Preheat oven to 350 degrees. Lightly grease a loaf pan-or a muffin tin. Mash the bananas in a mixing bowl. Then add the rest of ingredients and mix. Pour batter into prepared loaf and bake for one hour, or until toothpick comes out clean. For muffins reduce baking time. The bread will rise while in the oven, but will sink when taken out. Let the bread cool for fifteen minutes in the pan. This is necessary for the bread to set since it has no flour in it.

Reducing sugar in my diet is easy for me.

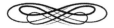

Kale

✓ Great detox food

✓ Anti-inflammatory food

✓ Filled with powerful antioxidants

✓ High in iron - essential in the formation of hemoglobin and enzymes for cell growth and proper liver function.

✓ Helps lower cholesterol levels

✓ High in vitamin C which supports our immune system

✓ Contains vitamin A which helps protect vision

✓ Great source of beta carotene

✓ Loaded with calcium

✓ Contains vitamins E and K, folate and magnesium

✓ High in fiber

Kale Salad with Avocados and Capers

Ingredients

1 bunch kale, rinsed and torn into bite-size pieces
1 ripe avocado, cubed
1 lemon, juiced
2 tablespoons capers, or to taste

Directions

Place kale in a salad bowl and pour enough lemon juice to adequately cover the greens."Massage" lemon juice and kale by hand, (the acid in the lemon breaks down the kale). Add the cubed avocado and capers to taste and mix together.

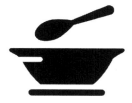

I am filled with gratitude for the blessings in my life.

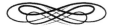

Kelp

✓ Assists in weight management and weight loss by improving metabolism and energy

✓ Helps in thyroid gland regulation with high levels of iodine

✓ Alkaline food which improves the body's pH level

✓ Helps remove radioactive particles and heavy metals from the body and is a blood purifier

✓ Helps with hydration and cancer prevention

✓ Helps relieve arthritis stiffness

✓ Contains 46 minerals, 16 amino acids and 11 vitamins

✓ High in calcium and magnesium which aid in strengthening bones and teeth

✓ Contains folic acid which can help protect blood vessels and decrease the risk of cardiovascular disease

Kelp Noodles and Sautéed Greens

Ingredients

1 onion, diced
2 tablespoon coconut oil
2 bunches greens (Choose: kale, Swiss chard, collard or beet greens)
1 12 – 16 oz. package kelp noodles, rinsed and cut with scissors
3 cloves garlic, crushed
Bragg's Liquid Aminos

Directions

Remove stems from all greens and wash. Slice greens into bite size pieces. Sauté onion in coconut oil. Add greens to sautéed onion and sauté until wilted. Add kelp noodles, garlic and Bragg's Liquid Aminos to taste.

My muscles love to move and exercise
keeps me youthful and healthy.

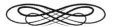

Kiwi

✓ High in immune boosting vitamin C

✓ High in potassium which helps manage blood pressure

✓ Contains enzymes to aid digestion

✓ Contains high level of lutein which protects against macular degeneration and other eye problems

✓ Contains antioxidant vitamin E which is great for the skin

✓ Helps create alkaline balance in the body

✓ Helps fight heart disease by helping reduce blood clotting

✓ Great source of fiber

Baked Salmon with Spinach and Strawberry Kiwi Salsa

Ingredients

4 (3-ounce) salmon fillets, skin removed
1 teaspoon lemon zest
1 lb. strawberries, diced
2 kiwi fruits, peeled and diced
1 cucumber, diced
1 jalapeño, seeded and minced
2 tablespoons chopped fresh mint leaves
2 tablespoons fresh lemon juice, divided
1 lb. baby spinach leaves, rinsed but not dried

Directions

Preheat oven to 350°F. Place salmon on a baking sheet and sprinkle with lemon zest. Bake 15 to 18 minutes or until cooked through.

Meanwhile, place strawberries, kiwi, cucumber, jalapeño, mint and 1 tablespoon lemon juice in a medium bowl and toss until combined. Set aside. Heat a large, high-sided skillet over medium heat. Add spinach, with water still clinging to leaves, cover and cook 5 minutes or until wilted, stirring occasionally. Stir in remaining lemon juice. Divide spinach among plates. Top with salmon and salsa and serve.

*Happiness fills me as I release that which
no longer benefits me.*

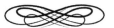

Lemons

✓ Great alkalizer for body - balances pH levels

✓ Excellent source of vitamin C to protect immune system

✓ Strengthens liver and helps flush out toxins, aid digestion and encourage bile production

✓ Reduce joint pain and inflammation by dissolving uric acid

✓ Contain potassium which helps nourish brain and nerve cells

✓ Help relieve colds, sore throats and coughs (in hot water)

✓ Prevent the formation of wrinkles and acne

✓ Help relieve constipation

✓ Strengthen the liver by providing energy to the liver enzymes

Lemon and Artichoke Chicken

This is a twist on chicken piccata using bone-in chicken.

4 Servings

Ingredients

4 tablespoons coconut oil, divided
¼ onion, sliced
2 cups artichoke hearts drained and rinsed
¼ cup capers, drained
Juice of 2 lemons
2 lbs. chicken pieces - with the bone
Sea salt and black pepper to taste

Directions

Preheat oven to 375F. In a large, oven-safe skillet over medium heat, melt 2 tablespoons of coconut oil. Add the onion and sauté until translucent. Add the artichoke hearts, capers, and lemon juice. Stir to combine. Place the chicken pieces in skillet and top each piece with the remaining 2 tablespoons coconut oil. Place the entire skillet into the oven for 45 minutes or until the chicken juices run clear when pierced with a knife.

Good health comes easily to me because I deserve it.

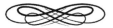

Lentils

✓ Contain high levels of soluble fiber to lower cholesterol

✓ Rich in protein (26% of calories are protein)

✓ Stabilize blood sugar

✓ Help prevent constipation

✓ Great source of folate and magnesium that support heart health

✓ Increase energy

"I feel that good food should be a right and not a privilege, and it needs to be without pesticides and herbicides. And everybody deserves this food. And that's not elitist."

- **Alice Waters**

Black Lentil Salsa Dip

This is one of my favorite quick, easy and simple appetizers that I turn to when I am short on time.

Ingredients

2 cups beluga black lentils (or use refrigerated cooked lentils)
1 16 oz. jar organic salsa

Directions

Cook lentils with four cups water for 20 – 25 minutes until soft and water is absorbed.

Cool lentils, then add salsa to desired taste. Serve with cut up vegetables or crackers.

As I increase my sleep, I am more relaxed, have more energy, and easily lose weight.

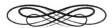

Mushrooms

✓ Contain potassium which helps control blood pressure

✓ Help keep blood sugar stable

✓ Dietary fiber which protects against heart disease

✓ Contain B vitamins which help break down proteins, fats and carbohydrates. Also promotes healthy skin and proper functioning of digestive and nervous systems

✓ Good source of minerals

✓ Rich source of selenium which protects body cells from damage

Spinach-Stuffed Mushrooms

6 Servings

Ingredients

20 medium mushrooms
¼ cup chopped shallots, scallions or onion
2 cloves garlic, chopped
1 tablespoon balsamic vinegar
½ teaspoon Bragg's Liquid Aminos
2 cups chopped fresh spinach
½ cup plain Greek yogurt
Salt and pepper to taste

Directions

Wash mushrooms and carefully remove the stems without breaking caps. Finely chop the stems. Combine the shallots, garlic and vinegar in a small skillet and cook for 1 to 2 minutes. Add chopped mushroom stems and Bragg Liquid Aminos and cook, stirring occasionally, for 3 to 5 minutes, until the mushrooms soften and release their juices. Add the spinach and cook, stirring until wilted and liquid in pan is absorbed. Remove from heat and let cool for a few minutes. Stir in yogurt and season with salt and pepper to taste.

Preheat the oven to 350ºF. Fill each mushroom cap with spinach mixture and place in a baking pan. Bake for 20 minutes until tender. Remove from oven and let stand for a few minutes allowing filling to set before serving.

*I have control over my eating habits
and I make healthy choices.*

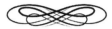

Oatmeal

✓ Lowers cholesterol by providing soluble fiber

✓ Reduces risk of high blood pressure and heart disease

✓ Contains antioxidants to fight off free radicals

✓ Stabilizes blood sugar

✓ Good source of magnesium which regulates the body's insulin and glucose levels which prevent diabetes

✓ Boosts immune system

✓ Helps with weight loss because fiber keeps you full longer

Apple-Berry Baked Oatmeal

This easy, baked breakfast dish is irresistibly rich and fragrant. Serve at brunch, or cut into slices and pack for breakfast to eat warm or cold.

Serves 8

Ingredients

Coconut oil cooking spray
2 cups frozen mixed berries
2 cups rolled oats
½ cup chopped pecans
1 teaspoon baking powder
½ teaspoon fine sea salt
1 cup applesauce
1 cup almond milk
½ cup Greek yogurt
1/3 cup maple syrup
2 teaspoons vanilla extract
1 egg plus 1 egg yolk

Directions

Preheat oven to 375°F. Oil a 9-inch pie pan with cooking spray; set aside. In a large bowl, stir together berries, oats, pecans, baking powder, salt and apple. In a medium bowl, whisk together milk, yogurt, syrup, vanilla, egg and extra yolk; stir into oat mixture. Transfer to prepared pan and bake until firm and golden brown on top, about 50 minutes. Cut into slices and serve.

*My pantry, refrigerator and freezer are filled
with health enhancing foods.*

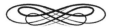

Onions

- ✓ Contain phytochemicals which improve vitamin C absorption resulting in improved immunity

- ✓ Contain chromium, which assists in regulating blood sugar

- ✓ Can reduce inflammation and helps heal infections

- ✓ Raw onion encourages the production of good cholesterol (HDL), which keeps your heart healthy

- ✓ Contain quercetin which aids in preventing cancer

- ✓ Can rid the body of free radicals

Roasted Root Vegetable Salad

Ingredients

Apple Cider Vinaigrette

3 tablespoons apple cider vinegar
1 tablespoon honey
¼ teaspoon sea salt
¼ teaspoon freshly ground black pepper
⅓ cup extra-virgin olive oil

Salad

1 medium red onion, cut into chunks
2 large carrots, halved, cut into ½ -inch pieces
2 large parsnips, halved lengthwise, cut into ½-inch pieces
1 medium rutabaga, peeled and cut into ½ inch pieces
2 tablespoons extra-virgin olive oil
¾ teaspoon herbs de Provence
¾ teaspoon kosher salt
½ teaspoon freshly ground black pepper
5 oz. bag of baby arugula
1 ripe pear, halved, cored, cut into thin wedges
½ cup chopped walnuts, toasted

Directions

Preheat oven to 400 degrees F. In a large bowl combine the red onion, carrots, rutabaga and parsnips. Add oil, herbs de Provence, salt and pepper; and toss to coat. Scatter the vegetables on a large baking sheet lined with parchment paper and roast until tender for 20 minutes, turning vegetables over once. Set aside.

Whisk the dressing ingredients together. In a salad bowl, combine the arugula, pear slices and roasted vegetables. Add the Apple Cider Vinaigrette and toss until coated. Sprinkle with chopped walnuts and serve.

I love my body and my life.

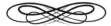

Pepitas (Pumpkin Seeds)

✓ High in omega-3 fatty acids, which decrease the body's ability to store fat

✓ High in protein which helps curb cravings and strengthen muscles

✓ Contain magnesium which protects heart health

✓ Rich source of zinc which is important for immunity, cell growth and division, sleep, mood, senses of taste and smell, eye and skin health, insulin regulation

✓ Supports prostate health

✓ Rich in healthy fats

✓ Contains tryptophan for restful sleep

✓ Has anti-inflammatory benefits

Southwestern Quinoa Salad

Serves 8

Ingredients

1 cup quinoa
1 cup pepitas (pumpkin seeds)
¼ cup chopped cilantro leaves
¼ cup lime juice
¾ teaspoon chili powder
1 15 oz. can black beans, rinsed and drained
2 tomatoes, finely chopped
1 zucchini, finely chopped
1 red bell pepper, chopped
1 cup fresh corn kernels - from 2 ears or 1 cup frozen corn
Salt and pepper to taste

Directions

Bring 2 cups water to a boil in a medium saucepan. Stir in quinoa, cover and cook until all water is absorbed about 10 minutes. Remove from heat and let stand 5 minutes. Fluff with a fork and let cool. Toss quinoa with remaining ingredients in a large bowl.

I listen to my body's needs for rest, relaxation, exercise, a hug or a good meal.

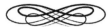

Pomegranates

✓ Very powerful anti-oxidants
✓ Potent anti-cancer and immune supporting effects
✓ Lower cholesterol and other cardiac risk factors
✓ Lower blood pressure

Extracting Seeds from Pomegranates

Cut the fruit into quarters. Submerge the quarters in a large bowl of cold water and place it in the kitchen sink to contain any squirting juice. Using your fingers, gently detach the seeds from the membrane and rind. The seeds will sink to the bottom of the bowl. Discard any pith, drain the water, blot the seeds lightly with paper towels.

Orange Avocado Salsa with Pomegranate Seeds

Makes about 4 cups

Ingredients

1 tablespoon fresh lime juice
1 teaspoon kosher or sea salt
1/8 teaspoon freshly ground black pepper
6 blood oranges
1 pomegranate
1 large Hass avocado, cut into ½-inch pieces
2/3 cup diced red onion
1 jalapeno, seeds and ribs removed, minced (optional)
2 green onions including green tops, cut in thin diagonal slices
¼ cup chopped fresh cilantro leaves

Directions

In a large bowl, whisk together lime juice, salt, and pepper until salt dissolves. Remove all skin, white pith, and seeds from the oranges, reserving any juice that's squeezed out in the process. Drain juice into a measuring cup and set aside. Cut orange segments into ½-inch pieces and add to bowl containing lime juice.

Remove seeds from pomegranates (see directions at left) and add to the orange segments.

Add the avocado, red onion, jalapeño, green onion, and cilantro. Using a rubber spatula, gently fold the ingredients together, being careful to not mash the avocados. Add reserved orange juice, 1 tablespoon at a time, until salsa is moist but not soupy. Taste and adjust seasoning. Transfer to a serving bowl, cover, and set aside for at least 1 hour to allow flavors to meld. Serve at room temperature with tortilla chips.

*I am a healthy-eating role model for
my family and friends.*

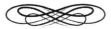

Pumpkin

- ✓ High in vitamin C
- ✓ Boosts the immune system
- ✓ High in vitamin A which supports good vision
- ✓ Contains beta carotene which supports eye health
- ✓ Contains fiber
- ✓ High in potassium
- ✓ Helps keep skin wrinkle free

Pumpkin Soup

This sweet and creamy soup has just a hint of spiciness. It can also be made with pureed winter squash, yams, or sweet potatoes in place of pumpkin.

Makes 2 quarts

Ingredients

1 tablespoon coconut oil
1 onion, chopped
2 garlic cloves, minced
½ teaspoon mustard seeds
½ teaspoon turmeric
½ teaspoon ground ginger
½ teaspoon ground cumin
¼ teaspoon cinnamon
¾ teaspoon salt
2 cups water or vegetable broth
1 15 oz. can of pumpkin
2 tablespoons maple syrup
1 tablespoon lemon juice
2 cups almond, coconut or hemp milk

Directions

Heat coconut oil in a large pot. Add onion and garlic and cook over medium heat until onion is soft, about 5 minutes. Add mustard seeds, turmeric, ginger, cumin, cinnamon, and salt and cook 2 minutes over medium heat, stirring constantly.

Whisk in water or broth, pumpkin, syrup or other sweetener, and lemon juice. Simmer 15 minutes. Remove from heat and stir in nondairy milk. Puree soup with immersion blender.

I walk in healing energy where ever I go.

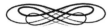

Quinoa

✓ Complete protein with all nine essential amino acids

✓ High in fiber

✓ Contains iron

✓ Gluten-free

✓ Contains magnesium to relax blood vessels and support formation of healthy bones and teeth

✓ Contains lysine which supports tissue growth and repair

✓ Contains riboflavin which improves energy metabolism

Quinoa Loaf with Mushrooms and Peas

Ingredients

1 tablespoon coconut oil
8 ounces button mushrooms, sliced
Salt and ground black pepper to taste
1 15 oz. can garbanzo beans, rinsed and drained
¾ cup rolled oats
2 cups cooked quinoa
1 cup frozen green peas
½ cup chopped fresh parsley
10 sundried tomatoes packed in oil, drained and chopped
1 cup chopped red onion

Directions

Preheat oven to 350°F. Lightly grease an 8-inch loaf pan with oil; set aside. Heat oil in a large skillet over medium-high heat; add mushrooms, salt and pepper and cook, stirring occasionally, until mushrooms are golden brown, 6 to 8 minutes.

Combine beans, oats and ½ cup water in a food processor and pulse until almost smooth. In a large bowl, combine mushrooms, bean mixture, quinoa, peas, parsley, tomatoes, onion, salt and pepper. Transfer mixture to prepared loaf pan, gently pressing down. Bake until firm and golden brown, 1 to 1¼ hours. Set aside to let rest for 10 minutes before slicing and serving.

*I pay attention to my thoughts because every cell
in my body responds to what I think.*

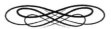

Red Bell Peppers

- ✓ Rich source of vitamins A and C

- ✓ Good source of fiber

- ✓ Powerful antioxidant

- ✓ Contain folate and vitamin K

- ✓ Loaded with nutrients and phytochemicals

- ✓ Contain lutein and zeaxanthin, which may slow the development of eye disease

- ✓ Contain lycopene, which decreases cancer risk

- ✓ Contain vitamin B6 which is a natural diuretic

Quinoa or Buckwheat Stuffed Peppers

Ingredients

2 cups cooked quinoa or buckwheat
1 tablespoon coconut oil
1 medium onion, chopped fine
4-6 cloves garlic, chopped fine
2 stalks celery, chopped fine
1 lb. greens such as kale, chopped
6 red bell peppers, seeded and parboiled 5 minutes
1 teaspoon sea salt or to taste
¾ teaspoon pepper
2 tablespoons dried basil
1 teaspoon cinnamon

Directions

Sauté onion in coconut oil and seasonings until translucent. Add celery, garlic, and kale, cook until tender. Combine quinoa with cooked vegetables; taste and adjust seasonings. Stuff peppers with quinoa mixture. Bake at 350 F degrees in an oiled casserole for 45 minutes.

Note: To cook quinoa, rinse quinoa several minutes in a strainer. Cook just like rice, using a two-to-one ratio of water to grain and a pinch of sea salt. Buckwheat is cooked in the same way.

My energy level is high and I feel great.

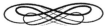

Salmon

- ✓ Excellent source of omega–3 fatty acids which help lower "bad" cholesterol and raise good cholesterol for heart health

- ✓ Contains vitamins A, B and D, plus calcium, iron, phosphorus and selenium

- ✓ Excellent protein source

- ✓ Helps lower blood pressure

- ✓ Helps prevent hardening of the arteries

- ✓ Protects nervous system from effects of aging

- ✓ Helps brain work better and supports memory improvement

- ✓ Helps lower blood sugar levels

Super Salmon Salad

When I attended the Institute of Integrative Nutrition in New York City to receive my training to be a Certified Health Coach 1200 students attended classes all day Saturday and Sunday. On Saturday evening 19 of us would climb up six flights of stairs to attend a fabulous cooking class in Andrea Beaman's (andreabeaman.com) apartment. This recipe is one of my many favorite recipes from her classes.

Ingredients

1 15 oz. can of wild salmon
½ red onion, diced small
¼ cup parsley, minced
1-2 stalks celery, diced
¼ cup olive oil
1 tablespoon Dijon mustard
1 teaspoon honey or agave nectar
2 tablespoon apple cider vinegar
Sea salt and pepper to taste

Directions

Drain salmon and place in mixing bowl. Combine with diced red onion, celery and parsley. Whisk together olive oil, mustard, honey, apple cider vinegar and sea salt and pepper to taste. Mix dressing with salmon salad. Eat spread on top of a collard green or romaine lettuce leaf or roll up as a wrap.

*I experience an abundance of energy
and vitality from eating greens.*

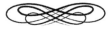

Spinach

✓ Contains vitamin A

✓ Source of phyto-nutrients that help prevent disease

✓ Contains potassium, copper, zinc, manganese, folate, magnesium
  and iron

✓ Contains vitamin K which helps strengthen bones

✓ Good source of soluble fiber which helps lower cholesterol

✓ Good source of anti-oxidant vitamins that protect against free
  radicals

✓ Contains vitamin C which helps develop immunity to infectious agents
  and free radicals

✓ Contains omega-3 fatty acids and B complex vitamins

Spinach, Beet, and Orange Salad with Ginger-Honey Dressing

Serves 2-4

Ingredients

2 small beets, scrubbed and trimmed
6 cups baby spinach
2 medium oranges, peeled and cut into sections

Dressing

4 tablespoons rice vinegar
2 tablespoons honey
1 teaspoon paprika
2 teaspoons grated fresh ginger
chili powder to taste
Juice of 1 lime

Directions

Boil beets until tender. Remove from heat, let cool to handle. Skins will easily peel off while still warm. Cut beets into bite-size wedges. Arrange spinach on a platter and top with beets and oranges.

To prepare the dressing:

Mix vinegar, honey, paprika, ginger, lime juice and chili powder and drizzle over spinach salad.

I am happy, healthy and joyful.

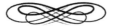

Sweet Potatoes

- ✓ Fight inflammation

- ✓ Contain vitamins A, B, C and D

- ✓ Contain antioxidants for disease protection

- ✓ Help stabilize blood sugar

- ✓ Contain potassium, beta-carotene and calcium

- ✓ Provide fiber to prevent constipation, lower cholesterol, and reduce acidity

- ✓ Help maintain skin's elasticity

- ✓ Contain magnesium for heart health and coping with stress

- ✓ Contain iron which is a carrier of oxygen and supports muscle and brain function

Sweet Potato and Tomato Soup

This soup recipe is from my friend, Lee Surwit, whose parents were friends with my mother in Poland. Lee received the recipe from her sister Zela. Lee and Zela's aunt and uncle introduced my parents in Germany after the Holocaust.

The recipe contains three vegetables that are high in beta-carotene: carrots, sweet potatoes and tomatoes.

4 Servings

Ingredients

1 tablespoon coconut oil
1 cup finely chopped onion
1 stalk celery, finely chopped
1 carrot, peeled and finely chopped
2 large sweet potatoes, peeled and diced
1 16 oz. can diced tomatoes
1 to 2 cups water
¼ teaspoon ground nutmeg
Salt and freshly ground black pepper
Chopped parsley (for garnish)

Directions

Heat the oil in a 4-quart pot over medium heat. Add the onion and celery. Sauté for 10 to 15 minutes until the celery has softened. Add the carrot and potatoes and sauté for 10 minutes more. Add the tomatoes and 1 to 2 cups of water or chicken broth and bring to a boil. Lower the heat, cover and cook for 30 to 35 minutes until the potatoes are tender. Using an immersion blender, puree but leave some chunks of vegetables in the soup. Add the nutmeg and continue cooking for 5 minutes. Taste and adjust seasonings. Garnish with chopped parsley.

I enjoy planning and organizing quick and easy meals.

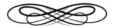

Tempeh

✓ Provides beneficial bacteria to the gut

✓ Helps flush out harmful toxins

✓ High in fiber

✓ Low in sodium

✓ Contains natural antibiotics

✓ Helps control blood sugar levels

✓ Easy to digest

Tempeh "Chicken" Salad

A vegetarian and vegan "chicken" salad recipe made with tempeh as a chicken substitute. To turn this tempeh salad into a curried tempeh salad, add raisins and slivered almonds and increase the amount of curry. This is one of those recipes that is best made ahead of time so it has plenty of time to chill in the refrigerator. This allows the tempeh to soak up all the flavors.

Ingredients

1 package tempeh, cut into ½ inch cubes
2 teaspoons mustard
2 tablespoons vegenaise
Juice of one lemon
2 teaspoons pickle relish
2 tablespoons green onion, minced
2 stalks celery, diced
¼ cup chopped parsley
½ red bell pepper, diced
¼ teaspoon curry powder (optional)
Dash of cayenne pepper (optional)
Sea salt and pepper to taste

Directions

In a pot or skillet, bring a few inches of water to a boil and add the tempeh. Allow to simmer covered for 15 minutes. Drain. Refrigerate tempeh until cool.

In a large bowl, combine the cooled tempeh with the remaining ingredients.

Enjoy your tempeh chicken salad on a bed of lettuce, between two lightly toasted pieces of bread, in a collard green wrap or stuffed into pita bread.

I am open and receptive to all good.

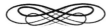

Tomatoes

✓ Contain antioxidant lycopene

✓ Help lower blood pressure

✓ Improve HDL cholesterol

✓ Help keep the body alkaline

✓ Contain phytochemicals

✓ Contain vitamins B and C

✓ Contain iron, potassium, chromium, biotin, lutein, and beta carotene

"The doctor of the future will no longer treat the human frame with drugs, but rather will cure and prevent disease with nutrition."

- Thomas Edison

Tomato Basil Soup

Ingredients

1 28 oz. can organic diced tomatoes
½ cup loosely packed basil leaves
1 tablespoon balsamic vinegar
2 teaspoons honey
Freshly ground pepper

Directions

Put all ingredients in food processor and pulse until blended. Chill and serve garnished with basil sprig and ground walnuts. You may also serve this soup warm.

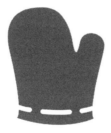

*Throughout the day I breathe deeply
to release any fear and tension.*

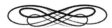

Turmeric

✓ Supports joint and muscle health

✓ Supports heart health

✓ Boosts detoxification

✓ Protects brain cells

✓ Is a natural mood enhancer

✓ Enhances weight loss

✓ Fights inflammation

✓ Promotes youthful and radiant skin

Red Lentil Soup with Lime

Ingredients

2 cups split red lentils, picked over and rinsed several times
1 tablespoon turmeric
3 tablespoons coconut oil
1 large onion, finely diced
2 teaspoons ground cumin
1 teaspoon mustard
1 bunch of cilantro, chopped
Juice of 3 limes
1 5 oz. bag of spinach, chopped small

Directions

Place the lentils in a soup pot with 2½ quarts water, turmeric, and 1 tablespoon of coconut oil. Bring to a boil, lower heat and simmer covered, until the lentils are soft and falling apart, about 20 minutes. Puree for a smooth and nicer looking soup.

While the soup is cooking, prepare the onion flavoring: In a medium skillet over low heat, cook the diced onion in 2 tablespoons of the remaining coconut oil with the cumin and mustard, stirring occasionally. When soft (about the time the lentils are cooked or after 15 minutes), add the cilantro and cook for 1 minute more. Add the onion mixture to the soup with the juice of 2 limes. Taste, and add more lime juice if needed to bring up the flavors. The soup should be a tad sour. Add the spinach at end of cooking and enjoy!

My health is vibrant and dynamic.

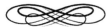

Walnuts

✓ May help reduce the risk of breast cancer

✓ Contain antioxidants that boost heart health and phytosterols

✓ Packed with omega-3 fatty acids which may help reduce depression, cancer, Alzheimer's disease and inflammatory diseases

✓ Reduce risk of diabetes

✓ Contain L-arginine which promotes healthy blood pressure

✓ Can help reduce stress

✓ Contain ellagic acid that helps support a healthy immune system

Vegetarian Mock Chopped Liver

Ingredients

3 onions, sliced
8 oz. frozen organic green beans
2 hard-boiled eggs
½ cup walnuts
Sea salt

Directions

Sauté onions in coconut or olive oil until caramelized. The longer the onions are cooked the tastier the "chopped liver" is. Steam green beans. Place all ingredients in a food processor and pulse so that the ingredients combine and look like "chopped liver" but not like a puree. Add salt to taste. Refrigerate for 1 hour to blend flavors. Serve with cut vegetables or crackers.

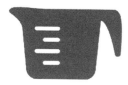

*My weight loss accelerates as I drink half
my body weight in water every day.*

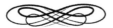

Water

- ✓ Energizes muscles
- ✓ Helps keep skin looking healthy
- ✓ Can help with weight loss
- ✓ Can help prevent constipation
- ✓ Flushes toxins out of the body
- ✓ Helps maintain body fluids balance of body fluids

Morning Elixer

Ingredients

1 cup warm or room temperature water
Juice from 1 lemon
1 teaspoon Bragg's raw apple cider vinegar 1 teaspoon raw honey OR
      a couple drops of stevia
½ teaspoon of cinnamon (optional)
(Use stevia if you are on a yeast cleansing diet or low sugar diet)

Stimulates digestion, releases toxins from the liver and jump-starts your digestive enzymes.

Health Benefits of Lemon Water

I am often asked: "What is one simple thing that I can do each day to improve my health?" Here it is:

Drink lemon water first thing in the morning!

Here are the reasons why:

1. Improves digestion

2. Boosts immune system

3. Hydrates your body

4. Boosts energy

5. Promotes healthy and rejuvenated skin

6. Reduces inflammation

7. Aids weight loss

8. Alkalizes your body

9. Has cleansing properties

10. Has antibacterial and antiviral properties

11. Reduces mucus And phlegm

12. Freshens breath

13. Boosts brain power

14. Has anti-cancer properties

15. Helps get you off caffeine or reduces the amount you drink

"It is never too late to be what you might have been."
- George Elliot

52 Tips, Tactics and Inspirations for Maintaining a Healthy Life

1. Take small steps at a time rather than trying to change everything at once.

2. Incorporate your changes into your daily life for 21 days, and it will become a habit.

3. Only make a couple of new changes every 21 days.

4. It doesn't matter when you start a new habit, just start.

5. Success depends on making a clear decision and then jumping into action.

6. We cannot go back and make a brand new start but we can start from now and make a brand new beginning.

7. End your day by writing down five things that you are grateful for and five things that went well during the day.

8. "Gratitude unlocks the fullness of life. It turns what we have into enough and more. It turns denial into acceptance, chaos into order and confusion to clarity. It can turn a meal into a feast, a house into a home and a stranger into a friend. Gratitude makes sense of our past, brings peace for today and creates a vision for tomorrow." - Melody Beattie

9. "The talent for being happy is appreciating what you have instead of what you don't have" – Woody Allen

10. As Deepak Chopra says: "Every time you are tempted to react in the same old way, ask yourself if you want to be a prisoner of the past or a pioneer of the future."

11. We are what we believe ourselves to be.

12. MISTAKES are: Meaningful Incidents Sure to Accelerate Knowledge, Exploration and Self-Awareness.

13. Life consists not in holding good cards, but in playing those you hold well.

14. Think of healthy eating as a way of life and not a diet.

15. It takes 21 days to change the chemistry of our body.

16. Eat real food not chemicals or processed food.

17. Start your day with 16 ounces of warm water with the juice of one-half lemon.

18. Drink water before your meal or after your meal because digestion begins in the mouth and we don't want to dilute our digestive juices.

19. To figure out how much water you need to drink, divide your body weight in half and drink that many ounces of water per day.

20. Dehydration appears as a sensation of hunger so drink water before eating something.

21. Eat breakfast within 45 minutes of getting up so your cells trust you and know they will be fed.

22. Have 15 grams or more of protein for breakfast.

23. Don't eat the same breakfast two days in a row because it's important to surprise our cells just the way we do when we vary a workout routine.

24. Buy plain Greek yogurt with 20 – 24 grams of protein.

25. Make your own fruit flavored yogurt by adding fresh or frozen organic berries or fruit juice sweetened jams.

26. To keep your blood sugar stabilized, eat a small amount of protein between meals.

27. Blood sugar stabilization helps with weight loss, maintains energy and helps with eliminating or subsiding cravings.

28. Keep peeled hard boiled eggs on hand for a quick boost of protein.

29. Instead of eating sugar for sweet cravings eat these sweet vegetables: corn, carrots, onions, beets, winter squashes, sweet potatoes, and yams.

30. To calculate the number of teaspoons of sugar in a serving, divide the grams of sugar by 4.

31. Sometimes cravings can be caused by a lack of what I call "primary food"—not food at all but a need for some fresh air, activity, a chat with a friend, creative expression or spiritual fulfillment. Check in with yourself to see what's missing.

32. Eat red radishes, daikon radish, green cabbage or burdock to reduce food cravings and maintain blood sugar levels.

33. Greens are one of the most important foods to eat because they support blood purification, improve circulation, strengthen your immune system, clear congestion and lift your spirits.

34. Cook a pot of soup each week and freeze extra containers so you always have a healthy, quick and easy meal.

35. When cooking fish or chicken always cook extra to have on hand for a salad or for a quick nibble of protein.

36. Every food has an energy associated with it.

37. To feel more grounded or relaxed eat root vegetables, sweet vegetables, meat, fish or beans.

38. Eating leafy greens, fruits, raw foods or chocolate will help you feel more energetic, flexible and creative.

39. If you are tense or anxious look at the amount of sugar, caffeine, nut butters and alcohol that you are consuming.

40. To feel more connected or harmonious eat organic foods, whole foods and local foods.

41. Purchase organic whenever possible but keep in mind that all food doesn't have to be organic. Look up the "Dirty Dozen" and the "Clean 15" online for the most current list of foods.

42. When eating alone, treat yourself like company and set the table.

43. Eat your meals without electronic distractions; unplug and focus on your food and how you feel.

44. Buy yourself fresh flowers to enjoy—not just for company!

45. Take time for yourself to sit down, relax for a few minutes and enjoy your meal and the result will be better digestion.

46. Invite a friend to your home and cook a healthy meal together.

47. Organize some healthy snacks to take with you when you are traveling or when you will be out for the day.

48. Two of the most important things in life cannot be bought—love and time.

49. Always remember that "Health is Wealth".

50. "Obstacles are those frightful things you see when you take your eyes off the goal." – Henry Ford.

51. Wisdom is knowing what to do next, skill is knowing how to do it, and virtue is doing it.

52. Just keep it simple and remember that you and your health are a top priority!

Using Affirmations to Create the Life You Want

Affirmations are the secret to creating the lives we want. This book gives you 52 affirmations to help you create the healthy lifestyle you want and deserve.

What are affirmations? Affirmations are statements about your intention or, in other words, what you want or intend to create in your life. All our thoughts—both positive and negative—are very powerful. We're creating our lives with our thoughts all the time—so we may as well do it consciously and get what we want rather than what we don't want.

What is it that you really want? For all of us, the life we want includes good health. Perhaps it's a habit or belief that you want to change or a quality you want to develop such as gratitude or inner peace. Whatever it is, your thoughts are the key and affirmations can help make it happen.

To create the life you want you need to stay focused on a positive vision rather than thinking about what you don't want. But there's more to it. If you constantly worry about things that might happen or think about what you don't want, you may actually be drawing those unwanted things to you. It's like an affirmation in reverse. That's why it's very important to be consciously aware of what you are thinking at all times.

Even though we know that staying positive is important, most of us are so busy that it's hard to stay aware of what we are thinking. Before we know it, we're concentrating on our fears rather than what we are hoping to create. Using affirmations calm and focus your mind and stop you from incessant worry.

How do affirmations work? It's really very simple. Whenever you are thinking about something you want—or something you don't want—you are sending out a signal. That signal is heard and responded to by your subconscious mind. What you are thinking affects you, other people and events. The fact is that you've been creating with your thoughts all your life even though you weren't aware of it!

Mixed Messages. Most of us send mixed messages. Let's say you are trying to create healthy eating habits. You try to stay focused on your vision, but sometimes you forget and think about junk food instead. You have sent a mixed signal. Mixed signals like this weaken our power to create. It's like rowing a boat in two directions at the same time. The more specific and consistent you are with your affirmations, the better they will work for you.

Writing Affirmations that Work. This book contains affirmations for each week of the year, but you may want to create your own as well. Affirmations are always written in first person and in present tense, as if whatever you want were already happening or had already come to pass. This is a wee bit tricky because you must imagine that you already have what you want to create.

Example: Let's say I wanted to lose weight. If I created an affirmation like, "I will lose 25 pounds," I would have sent the wrong signal. "I will lose 25 pounds," tells my subconscious mind that I want something to happen in the future. The future, however, could be next month, next year or even the next decade!

So I would create a different affirmation, one written in present tense: "I maintain my optimum weight of 120 pounds easily and effortlessly." Do you see the difference? In this case, I have affirmed that I have already lost the weight. Because my subconscious doesn't know the difference between my thoughts and reality, it will begin to act as if I am already at my optimum weight. I will be creating what I am affirming, here and now. This technique may sound awkward at first, but keeping your affirmations in the present tense is essential!

Changing a Belief or Attitude. You can also use affirmations to help you change an attitude or belief. For instance, you might want to become more self-assured. You could use an affirmation like, "I am confident, and it shows in all that I do." You are affirming that you are confident in the present tense—right now. Since your subconscious believes every thought you think, you will soon find yourself feeling more self-confident and acting that way too. Because you now have begun to act more self-assured, people around you will begin to relate to you differently. You will not only have changed yourself, but you will have changed the people around you as well!

Staying Positive. It's important that your affirmations be written in a positive form. Let's say you wanted to change your habit of snacking on junk food. Rather than writing "I don't eat junk food," which includes the negative word "don't," write "I eat only foods that are healthy for me."

As you create your affirmations, you can be as specific as possible but very general affirmations work too. Here's an effective one that was first used nearly 100 years ago:

"Every day in every way I am getting better and better."

This or Something Better. Even though you think you know what you want, there might be something even better in store for you! Always keep the thought, "This or something better is happening for the highest purpose of all concerned," when you use affirmations. That way, you leave open the door to something even more desirable than what you might have imagined.

Energizing Your Affirmations. If you can, say your affirmations aloud. At the same time, create a picture in your mind of what your life looks like when you have what you are affirming. Adding other senses to your thoughts will strengthen the power of your affirmations. See, hear, smell, and touch whatever it is you desire in your mind.

Imagine the feeling you will have when what you are affirming becomes real. Feel the energy of those positive emotions in your body. The more clearly you can "experience" what you want in your mind, the more powerful your affirmations will be.

You can enhance the effectiveness of your affirmations by repeating them as you go to sleep. The more relaxed you are when you say them, the deeper they will sink into your psyche. The more you say your affirmations with sincerity, interest and faith, the faster they will work.

Dealing with Negative Thoughts. As you use your affirmations, negative thoughts may come up—"That's not reality!" or "I don't deserve that." This is normal. Just acknowledge the thought, then let it go. Breathe deeply and relax, then go back to your affirmation. As you become more comfortable with using affirmations, you'll find you have fewer and fewer negative thoughts.

 Writing affirmations isn't the hardest part. Remembering to use them is the most difficult part—and affirmations only work if you use them. Create reminders such as index cards propped up in your kitchen or on your desk.

Along with a healthy diet and exercise, changing your thinking will help you create optimal health. Best wishes to you as you create your life the way you've always wanted it to be!

"You are the sum total of everything you've ever seen, heard, eaten, smelled, been told, forgot - it's all there. Everything influences each of us, and because of that I try to make sure that my experiences are positive."

- Maya Angelou

My Own Affirmations

My Own Healthy Tips and Ideas

Notes

ABOUT THE AUTHOR

Freddi Pakier was a top-producing real estate broker in Tucson and a leader in the volunteer community for over 20 years. After observing declining health in loved ones and work associates, Freddi made a conscious decision to jump off-the-treadmill and follow her passion of promoting health and wellness which she had been studying for 30 years.

Freddi began her health coaching practice in 2007. She works with people in all walks of life and ages with a variety of health challenges and concerns.

Freddi holds a bachelors degree in Business and Education from Roosevelt University, a certification in Health Coaching from the Institute of Integrative Nutrition and Columbia University, and a certification from the American Association of Drugless Practitioners. She lives in North County San Diego, California.

Freddi is a nurturing wellness coach, an inspiring speaker, and a cooking instructor. She is a visiting chef at the Rancho La Puerta Spa in Tecate, Mexico.

FreddiPakier.com

$18.00

ISBN 978-0-692-44110-7

51800>